Table of Contents

What is systemic lupus erythematosus?

Systemic lupus erythematosus (SLE), commonly referred to simply as lupus, is a chronic autoimmune disease that can cause swelling (inflammation) and pain throughout your body. When you have an autoimmune disease, your body's immune system fights itself. The immune system is supposed to fight possible threats to the body — infections, for example — but, in this case, it goes after healthy tissue.

If you have lupus, you might experience joint pain, skin sensitivities and rashes, and issues with internal organs (brain, lungs, kidneys and heart). Many of your symptoms might come and go in waves — often called flare-ups. At times, symptoms of lupus might be mild or not noticeable (meaning they're in remission). Other times, you could experience severe symptoms of the condition that heavily impact your daily life.

The immune system normally fights off dangerous infections and bacteria to keep the body healthy. An autoimmune disease occurs when the immune system attacks the body because it confuses it for something foreign. There are many autoimmune diseases, including systemic lupus erythematosus (SLE).

The term lupus has been used to identify a number of immune diseases that have similar clinical presentations and laboratory features, but SLE is the most common type of lupus. People are often referring to SLE when they say lupus.

SLE is a chronic disease that can have phases of worsening symptoms that alternate with periods of mild symptoms. Most people with SLE are able to live a normal life with treatment.

According to the Lupus Foundation of America, at least 1.5 million Americans are living with diagnosed lupus. The foundation believes that the number of people who actually have the condition is much higher and that many cases go undiagnosed.

What are the different types of lupus?

There are several different types of lupus. Systemic lupus erythematosus is the most common. Other types of lupus include:

Cutaneous lupus erythematosus: This type of lupus affects the skin — cutaneous is a term meaning skin. Individuals with cutaneous lupus erythematosus may experience skin issues like a sensitivity to the sun and rashes. Hair loss can also be a symptom of this condition.

Drug-induced lupus: These cases of lupus are caused by certain medications. People with drug-induced lupus may have many of the same symptoms of systemic lupus erythematosus, but it's usually temporary. Often, this type of lupus goes away once you stop the medication that's causing it.

Neonatal lupus: A rare type of lupus, neonatal lupus is a condition found in infants at birth. Children born with neonatal lupus have antibodies that were passed to them from their mother — who either had lupus at the time of the pregnancy or may have the condition later in life. Not every baby born to a mother with lupus will have the disease.

Recognizing potential symptoms of SLE

Symptoms can vary and can change over time. Common symptoms include:

- severe fatigue
- joint pain
- joint swelling
- headaches
- a rash on the cheeks and nose, which is called a "butterfly rash"

- hair loss
- anemia
- blood-clotting problems

fingers turning white or blue and tingling when cold, which is known as Raynaud's phenomenon
Other symptoms depend on the part of the body the disease is attacking, such as the digestive tract, the heart, or the skin.

Lupus symptoms are also symptoms of many other diseases, which makes diagnosis tricky. If you have any of these symptoms, see your doctor. Your doctor can run tests to gather the information needed to make an accurate diagnosis.

Causes of SLE

The exact cause of SLE isn't known, but several factors have been associated with the disease.

Genetics

The disease isn't linked to a certain gene, but people with lupus often have family members with other autoimmune conditions.

Environment

Environmental triggers can include:

- ultraviolet rays
- certain medications
- viruses
- physical or emotional stress

- trauma
- Sex and hormones

SLE affects women more than men. Women also may experience more severe symptoms during pregnancy and with their menstrual periods. Both of these observations have led some medical professionals to believe that the female hormone estrogen may play a role in causing SLE. However, more research is still needed to prove this theory.

How is SLE diagnosed?

Your doctor will do a physical exam to check for typical signs and symptoms of lupus, including:

- sun sensitivity rashes, such as a malar or butterfly rash
- mucous membrane ulcers, which may occur in the mouth or nose
- arthritis, which is swelling or tenderness of the small joints of the hands, feet, knees, and wrists
- hair loss
- hair thinning

signs of cardiac or lung involvement, such as murmurs, rubs, or irregular heartbeats

No one single test is diagnostic for SLE, but screenings that can help your doctor come to an informed diagnosis include:

- blood tests, such as antibody tests and a complete blood count
- a urinalysis
- a chest X-ray

Your doctor might refer you to a rheumatologist, which is a doctor who specializes in treating joint and soft tissue disorders and autoimmune diseases.

Treatment for SLE

No cure for SLE exists. The goal of treatment is to ease symptoms. Treatment can vary depending on how severe your symptoms are and which parts of your body SLE affects. The treatments may include:

- anti-inflammatory medications for joint pain and stiffness, such as these options available online
- steroid creams for rashes
- corticosteroids to minimize the immune response
- antimalarial drugs for skin and joint problems
- disease modifying drugs or targeted immune system agents for more severe cases

Talk with your doctor about your diet and lifestyle habits. Your doctor might recommend eating or avoiding certain foods and minimizing stress to reduce the likelihood of triggering symptoms. You might need to have screenings for osteoporosis since steroids can thin your bones. Your doctor may also recommend preventive care, such as immunizations that are safe for people with autoimmune diseases and cardiac screenings,

Long-term complications of SLE

Over time, SLE can damage or cause complications in systems throughout your body. Possible complications may include:

- blood clots and inflammation of blood vessels or vasculitis
- inflammation of the heart, or pericarditis
- a heart attack
- a stroke
- memory changes
- behavioral changes
- seizures
- inflammation of lung tissue and the lining of the lung, or pleuritis
- kidney inflammation
- decreased kidney function
- kidney failure

SLE can have serious negative effects on your body during pregnancy. It can lead to pregnancy complications and even miscarriage. Talk with your doctor about ways to reduce the risk of complications.

Natural Remedies for Treating Lupus

Omega-3 Fatty Acids

Shown to curb inflammation, omega-3 fatty acids have been found to improve symptoms in lupus patients in several studies.You can increase your omega-3 intake by eating oily fish (such as salmon and sardines) or flaxseeds, or by taking a daily omega-3 supplement.

Herbal Medicine

Though not specifically studied in lupus patients, anti-inflammatory herbs like ginger and turmeric may be especially helpful for lupus patients suffering from arthritic symptoms.

Vitamin and Mineral Supplements

Corticosteroids (inflammation-fighting drugs often used in lupus treatment) may thin your bones and increase your risk of osteoporosis. To keep your bones strong while on corticosteroids, ask your healthcare provider about daily vitamin D and calcium supplements.

Mind-Body Therapies

Using mind-body techniques like hypnotherapy and guided imagery may help you deal with the stress of lupus.For more help in coping and alleviating stress, make sure to get plenty of sleep and exercise regularly. Ask your healthcare provider about the right amount and types of exercise for you.

DHEA

Research suggests that dehydroepiandrosterone (DHEA), a steroid hormone essential to the production of estrogen and testosterone) may enhance quality-of-life for people with lupus.

While DHEA shows promise as a complementary treatment for lupus, regular use of DHEA supplements could raise your risk of heart attack and some types of cancer. Therefore, it's critical to use DHEA only under the supervision of your primary care provider.

Diet Tips for Systematic Lupus Erythematosus

Despite what you might have read, there's no established diet for lupus. Just as with any medical condition, you should aim to eat a healthy blend of foods, including fresh fruits, vegetables, whole grains, legumes, plant fats, lean proteins, and fish.

However, certain foods may be better than others for managing your symptoms. Keep reading to find out what to include in your diet.

Switch from red meat to fatty fish

Red meat is full of saturated fat, which can contribute to heart disease. Fish are high in omega-3s. Try to eat more:

- salmon

- tuna

- mackerel

- sardines

Omega-3s are polyunsaturated fatty acids that help protect against heart disease and stroke. They can also reduce inflammation in the body.

Get more calcium-rich foods

The steroid drugs you may take to control lupus can thin your bones. This side effect makes you more vulnerable to fractures. To combat fractures, eat foods that are high in calcium and vitamin D. These nutrients strengthen your bones.

Calcium-rich foods include:

- low-fat milk

- cheese

- yogurt

- tofu

- beans

- calcium-fortified plant milks

- dark green leafy vegetables such as spinach and broccoli

Ask your doctor about taking a supplement if you're not getting enough calcium and vitamin D from food alone.

Limit saturated and trans fats

Everyone's goal should be to eat a diet that's low in saturated and trans fats. This is especially true for people with lupus. Steroids can increase your appetite and cause you to gain weight, so it's important to watch what you eat.

Try to focus on foods that will fill you up without filling you out, such as raw vegetables, air-popped popcorn, and fruit.

Avoid alfalfa and garlic

Alfalfa and garlic are two foods that probably shouldn't be on your dinner plate if you have lupus. Alfalfa sprouts contain an amino acid called L-canavanine. Garlic contains allicin, ajoene, and thiosulfinates, which can send your immune system into overdrive and flare up your lupus symptoms.

People who've eaten alfalfa have reacted with muscle pain and fatigue, and their doctors have noted changes on their blood test results.

Skip nightshade vegetables

Although there isn't any scientific evidence to prove it, some people with lupus find that they're sensitive to nightshade vegetables. These include:

- white potatoes
- tomatoes
- sweet and hot peppers
- eggplant

Keep a food diary to record what you eat. Eliminate any foods, including vegetables, that cause your symptoms to flare up every time you eat them.

Watch your alcohol intake

The occasional glass of red wine or beer isn't restricted. However, alcohol can interact with some of the medicines you take to control your condition. Drinking while taking NSAID drugs such as ibuprofen (Motrin) or naproxen (Naprosyn), for example, could increase your risk of stomach bleeding or ulcers. Alcohol can also reduce the effectiveness of warfarin (Coumadin) and may increase the potential liver side-effects of methotrexate.

Pass on salt

Set aside the saltshaker and start ordering your restaurant meals with less sodium. Here are some tips:

- order your sauces on the side, they are often high in sodium
- ask for your entrée to be cooked without added salt

- order an extra side of vegetables, which are rich in potassium

Eating too much salt can raise your blood pressure and increase your risk for heart disease, while potassium can help combat high blood pressure. Lupus already puts you at higher risk for developing heart disease.

Substitute other spices to enhance food flavor, such as:

- lemon
- herbs
- pepper
- curry powder
- turmeric

A number of herbs and spices have been sold on the web as lupus symptom relievers. But there is very little evidence that any of them work.

These products can interact with drugs you're taking for lupus and cause side effects. Don't take any herbal remedy or supplement without first talking to your doctor.

Top 5 tips for exercising with Lupus

Listen to your body. Exercise when your symptoms are minimal. It is important for you to be an expert of your own body and know what you can tolerate. If your body is not feeling up for it, then rest is the key.

Plan your exercise appropriately. Try and perform exercise on a day/time when you know you can get an adequate rest afterwards. Physical stress and exhaustion can trigger flares so it is important to ensure your body is getting a good recovery. Fatigue can be a problem for people with lupus, so it's important to pace yourself during exercise. It's okay to take breaks and rest accordingly, but don't give up altogether.

Vary your exercise. Try & get a complete range of exercises into your weekly routine to ensure you are utilising all systems effectively. Using different muscle groups and various body systems on different days can help your full body get a regular workout without overdoing it on one particular day. i.e. Cardiorespiratory (walking, bike, swimming) for good heart & lung health, Strength (weights) for good muscle & bone health, Mobility (yoga, stretching) for joint range of motion, & joint support, and Relaxation (mediation, rest) for stress & overall wellbeing.

Think carefully when exercising outdoors. Avoid outdoor exercise in the sun (particularly during high UV time from 11am-4pm in summer) because sunlight can trigger flares. Cover up by wearing a hat, long-sleeved shirts, and long pants, and use sunscreens with a sun protection factor of at least 30 if you walk/run or bike outdoors.

Start gradually and build up slowly. Starting with too much or increasing too ⁨quickly⁩ can bring on symptoms. Use the 10% rule to gauge how much to increase, that is, increase the duration and intensity of your workout by 10% per week. For example, increase by one minute if you walk for 10 minutes. Again, remember that each day may feel afferent for you so again it is important to read your body and have adjustments made accordingly.

Recipes for Systematic Lupus Erythematosus

1. Roasted Red Pepper And Feta Quinoa Salad

Ingredient

- 1 Tbsp. olive oil
- 1 Small onion, chopped
- 2 Cloves garlic, minced
- 2 Roasted red peppers,
- cut into bite sized pieces
- 1 Cup quinoa, rinsed
- 2 Cups vegetable broth
- 1 Tsp. dried oregano
- Salt & pepper to taste
- ½ Cup chickpeas
- ¼ Cup feta, crumbled
- ¼ Cup balsamic vinaigrette

Instruction

- Heat the oil in a pan.
- Add the onion and sauté until tender, about 5 to 7 minutes.
- Add the garlic and sauté until fragrant, about a minute.
- Add the roasted red peppers, Quinoa, vegetable broth and oregano Season with salt and pepper and bring to a boil.
- Reduce heat, cover, and simmer until the Quinoa is tender and the liquid has been absorbed, about 15 minutes.
- Remove from heat and mix in the chickpeas, feta and balsamic vinaigrette.

2. Date Bites

Ingredients

- 2 Cups dates

- ¾ cup raw sunflower seeds
- ¾ cup raw pumpkin seeds
- Cinnamon
- 2 Tbsp. shredded coconut
- 1 to 3 Tbsp. hemp seeds
- 2 to 4 Tbsp. chia seeds
- A dash of himalayan pink salt

Instruction

- Gather all the ingredients and place in a blender.
- Add a small amount of water to help with the blending, if necessary.
- Roll into balls, place them stacked in a mason jar and freeze.

3. **Chicken Tortilla Soup**

Ingredients

- 1 Onion, chopped
- 3 Cloves garlic, minced
- 1 Tbsp. olive oil
- 2 Tsp. chili powder
- 1 Tsp. dried cumin
- 1 (28 oz.) Can crushed tomatoes
- 1 (10.5 oz.) Can chicken broth
- 1¼ Cups water
- 1 Cup whole corn kernels, frozen
- 1 (4 oz.) Can chopped green chili peppers
- 1 (15 oz.) Can black beans, drained
- and rinsed
- 1/3 Cup chopped fresh cilantro
- 2 Boneless chicken breast halves, cooked
- and cut into bite-sized pieces
- Salt & pepper as needed

Optional toppings: Tortilla strips/chips,
- shredded mexican blend or other cheese,

- avocado slices, sour cream, chopped
- green onion

Instruction

- In a Dutch oven or medium stock pot heat oil over medium heat. Sauté onion and garlic in oil
- until soft. Stir in chili powder and cumin and cook until fragrant, about 30 to 45 seconds.
- Add tomatoes, broth, and water. Bring to a boil and simmer for 5 to 10 minutes.
- Stir in corn, chilis, beans, cilantro, and chicken. Simmer for 15 minutes.
- Ladle soup into individual serving bowls, and top with crushed tortilla strips, avocado slices,
- cheese, sour cream and chopped green onion.
- Note: Chicken can be cooked (cut into bite-sized pieces) in the same pot with some oil first,

- then removed before continuing with instructions above.

4. Broccoli leek soup

Ingredients
- 1 Large bunch broccoli
- (about 1 ½ pounds)
- 1 Tbsp. olive oil
- 1 Tbsp. unsalted butter (or vegan butter)
- 2 Medium leeks, white and light green
- parts only, thinly sliced
- 1 Medium baking potato, peeled and cut
- into 1-inch pieces
- 1 Clove garlic, thinly sliced
- 3 Cups low-sodium chicken or
- vegetable broth
- ¾ Tsp. salt
- pinch freshly ground pepper

- ¼ Cup half-and-half (optional)
- ¼ Cup snipped chives

Ingredients

- Separate broccoli stems from florets. Using a vegetable peeler, peel stems to remove tough outer layer, then slice into ¼-inch-thick circles. Break or cut the florets into small pieces. Reserve stems and florets separately.
- In a medium saucepan, heat oil and butter over medium heat. Add leeks and cook, stirring often, until softened and fragrant, about 3 minutes. Add broccoli stems, potato, and garlic, and cook 2 to 3 minutes. Add 3 cups water, broth, salt, and pepper; bring to
- a boil. Reduce heat; cover partially and simmer until broccoli and potato are tender, about 12 minutes.

- Add florets; bring to a boil and then simmer 5 minutes. Use an immersion blender in the pot or transfer soup in batches to a blender or food processor, and puree until smooth.
- Return soup to saucepan; add half-and-half if using and chives and reheat briefly

5. Tangy Glutenfree Pasta Salad

Ingredient
- ½ Box gluten-free penne pasta
- ½ Cup manzanilla olives
- 1 Cup cherry tomatoes
- 1 Packet Goya salad & vegetable
- seasoning
- 2 Tbsp. Italian seasoning
- 2 Tbsp. balsamic vinegar
- 2 Tbsp. extra virgin olive oil
- black pepper & salt to taste

Directions.

- Prepare penne pasta according to instructions on box (boil until al dente with a dash of salt and olive oil) then drain. Place in a large mixing bowl.

- Cut olives into halves. Cut cherry tomatoes in quarters. Add olives and tomatoes to bowl with pasta.

- Add Goya salad & vegetable seasoning, Italian seasoning, olive oil, balsamic vinegar, and a dash of black pepper to taste.

- Mix well with a spoon, then serve warm or chilled.

6. Chicken Zucchini Poppers

Ingredients

- 1 Pound ground chicken breast
- 2 Cups grated zucchini (leave peel on and

- squeeze out liquid with paper towels or a
- clean kitchen towel)
- 2 to 3 Green onions, sliced
- 3 to 4 Tbsp. cilantro, minced
- 1 Clove garlic, minced
- 1 Tsp. salt
- ½ Tsp. pepper
- ¾ Tsp. cumin (optional)
- Optional (if pan-frying): Avocado oil,
- coconut oil or ghee for cooking

Directions

- In a large bowl, mix together chicken, zucchini, green onion, cilantro, garlic, salt, pepper, and cumin (if using). Mixture will be quite wet.
- Scoop mixture with a small scoop or heaped tbsp. and gently smooth with your hands to get 20 to 24 poppers.
- To cook on the stovetop:

Heat a drizzle of oil in a medium pan over medium-low heat. Cook 4 to 5 at a time for about

5 to 6 minutes on the first side. Flip and cook an additional 4 to 5 minutes, or until golden brown and the centers are cooked through.

- To bake:

Preheat oven to 400 degrees. Drizzle olive or avocado oil onto a baking sheet lined with foil.

Bake for 15 to 20 minutes, or until cooked through. If desired, place under the broiler for an

additional 2 to 3 minutes or until browned on top.

- Serve with guacamole, salsa, or your favorite dip.

7. Summer Chickpea Salad

Ingredients

- 2 Cans of chickpeas, drained
- 2 Cucumbers, peeled, seeds
- removed and diced
- ½ Red onion, diced
- 1 Cup Italian parsley, chopped
- 4 Tbsp. olive oil
- 4 Tsp. red wine vinegar
- Crumbled feta to taste
- Salt/pepper to taste

Directions

- Combine all ingredients. Refrigerate for 2 hours to allow flavors to meld.

8. Peas Dips

Ingredients

- 1 Cup frozen peas
- 1 Small avocado
- ¼ Cup olive oil extra virgin
- 1 Tbsp. lemon juice
- Pinch of salt
- Fresh mint leaves

Directions

- Add all ingredients to a blender and blend until all ingredients are
well integrated.

Notes:

Blend the fresh mint leaves with all the ingredients or chop them and put it
as decoration on the dip.

Lighten the dip and convert it to a sauce by adding water to the mixture or

substituting the olive oil with plain yogurt.

Use it as dressing for your salads, burgers, falafel, etc.

9. Vegan Curry

Ingredient

- 2 Tsp. salt, for water
- 1 Pound sweet potato, cut into 1-inch cubes
- 1 Pound butternut squash, cut into 1-inch cubes
- 1 Tbsp. vegetable oil
- 1 Medium onion, diced
- 4 Cloves garlic, minced
- 2 Tsp. cumin
- 4 Tsp. curry powder
- 1 Tsp. salt

- 1 Tsp. black pepper
- 2 Centimeter pieces ginger, minced
- 1 Can diced tomatoes
- 1 Can chickpeas, drained
- 1 Can coconut milk

Directions

- Place sweet potatoes and squash into a large pot or dutch oven and cover with well-salted water. Bring to a boil, then reduce heat to a simmer, cover and let the potatoes cook until softer, about 10 minutes. Once cooked, drain the potatoes and set them aside.
- Return the pot to the stove and add 1 tbsp. of oil. Add onion and garlic and sauté over medium heat until onion is tender and starts to turn translucent, about 3 to 5 minutes.

- Add cumin, curry powder, salt, pepper and ginger. Stir to combine before adding tomatoes and chickpeas.
- Increase heat to medium-high and stir in the coconut milk. Bring to a simmer before adding the potatoes back to the pot. Reduce heat to low and cook everything together for 3 to 5 minutes before serving.
- Serve with basmati or jasmine rice.

10. Maqluba

Ingredients
- 2 ½Cups basmati rice
- 2 Tbsp. olive oil
- 1 Large onion, chopped
- 1 Pound minced beef or lamb
- 1 Tsp. allspice
- 1 Tsp. salt

- Coarsely crushed black pepper
- 3 1/3 Cups chicken stock hot
- 1 Small cauliflower, chopped into to bite
- sized pieces and roasted or grilled
- 1 Large eggplant, cubed
- 1 Zucchini, cubed
- 1 Red bell pepper, cubed
- tomatoes, sliced in rings
- 4 Pine nuts and parsley

Directions

- Rinse and drain the rice and set aside.
- Heat the olive oil in the saucepan over medium heat. Sauté the onions for about 3 to 4 minutes.
- Add meat, allspice, salt and ¼ tsp. pepper. Stir and brown the meat all over and cook for about 10 minutes on medium high heat. Try to

eliminate as much of the liquid from the beef as possible.

- Grease your saucepan of choice and layer in all of the tomatoes. Season with salt and pepper.
- Add the meat, pack it in, flatten, and season with salt and pepper. Repeat with vegetables and rice.
- Take a small saucer or back of a large spoon and place it face down on the rice and pour all the stock to prevent a gap or hole appearing in the rice.
- Place the pot on the stovetop, turn the heat on high for about 3 minutes to bring everything up to simmering point and the edges are bubbling.
- Put the lid on, turn the heat down and cook for about 45 minutes. If you think the rice isn't done, cook another 5 to 10 minutes.
- Take a large plate or serving platter, place it over the pot, and turn it upside down, inverting

the rice onto the platter, similar to a Spanish Tortilla. Once inverted, scatter with pine nuts and parsley and serve.

Nutritionist says:

• To reduce the fat: After sautéing the onions, add the meat and cook until browned.

Do not add spices yet. Once the meat has cooked, drain the meat in a colander and

run warm water over the meat to help drain the excess fat. Put the rinsed meat

back in the pan and then add the spices.

• To reduce the salt, wait until the end to season the dish with salt.

11. Rosemary Kale Chicken Soup

Ingredients

• 2 Qts. chicken broth (organic,

- low sodium or homemade)
- 1 Garlic clove, minced
- ½ Medium yellow onion, diced
- 2 Celery stalks, chopped
- 2 Cups chopped kale
- 1 Small sprig rosemary, stem
- removed, finely chopped
- 1 Cup cooked chicken
- Sea salt to taste
- Freshly ground pepper to taste

Directions

- Place all ingredients in a large pot over medium-high heat.
- Bring to a boil.
- Turn heat to low and simmer, covered, until veggies are tender,
- about 30 minutes.
- Add sea salt and pepper to taste

12. Avocado Toast With Cheese And Berries

Ingredients

- 1 Piece of any kind whole
- grain bread
- ½ Large avocado, ripe
- handful of berries
- 1 Oz. hard cheese, thinly sliced
- Optional: Honey

Directions

- Toast the bread then remove the avocado from the skin and place on
  top of bread. Use your fork to mash the avocado on top of the bread.
- Add a handful of berries and a few pieces of thinly sliced hard cheese.
- Finish off with a drizzle of honey

13. Slow Cooker Mushroom Rice

Ingredients

- 3 Tbsp. butter, divided
- 1 Pound cremini mushrooms, sliced
- 1 Yellow onion diced
- 2 Cloves garlic minced
- ½ Tsp. kosher salt
- ¼ Tsp. coarse ground pepper
- ½ Tsp. dry thyme
- 2 Cups rice
- 4 Cups vegetable or beef broth

Directions

- In heavy bottomed pot add 2 tbsp. butter and mushrooms.
- Cook on medium high for 3 to 5 minutes or until they start to caramelize.
- Stir and cook an additional 3 minutes.

- Remove the mushrooms and put them into slow cooker.
- Add in onions, salt, pepper and thyme along with the last tbsp. of butter and cook on
- medium for 3 to 5 minutes or until they start to turn golden brown.
- Add in garlic, stir and cook for 1 minute.
- Scrape the onion garlic mixture into the slow cooker.
- Add in rice and broth.
- Cook on high for 2 hours.

14. Dairy-Sensitive Bolognese

Ingredients
- 1 Tbsp. olive oil
- 3 Tbsp. butter or vegetable
- spread + 1 tbsp. for tossing pasta
- ½ diced onion

- 2 to 3 Cup diced celery, 3-4 ribs
- 2 to 3 Cup diced carrot
- ½ Cup pancetta
- ¾ Pound ground beef
- Salt and pepper
- 1 Cup unsweetened oat or
- almond milk
- 1 to 8 Tsp. ground nutmeg
- 1 Cup white wine, or red if
- necessary, or substitute
- chicken broth
- 2 Cups of canned San Marzano
- tomatoes, or any canned
- plum tomato
- 1 Pound pappardelle pasta
- A few sprigs of fresh oregano
- Freshly grated parmigianoreggiano or parmesan cheese
- for garnish

Directions

- Add oil and 3 tbsp. of butter or vegetable spread to a large pot
  on medium.

- Once the butter is melted, add the onion and stir occasionally until
  translucent. Add diced celery, carrot, and pancetta and cook for
  about 2 to 3 minutes or until the pancetta is light brown and
  slightly crispy.

- Add the ground beef and generously salt and pepper and cook until
  the meat is no longer pink while breaking up with a spoon.

- Add oat or almond milk, stir frequently and cook until there is almost
  no liquid left in the bottom of the pot.

- Add nutmeg and stir the beef mixture for 1 minute. Add the wine, stir and cook until there is

  almost no liquid left in the bottom of the pot.
- Open the can of tomatoes and with a knife or your hands break up or cut the tomatoes until there are no large pieces of tomato visible. Add 2 cups of tomatoes with the juice they came in. Bring the pot to a bubble and immediately turn the heat as low as the stove allows.
- The sauce should take about 15 minutes to bring down to a slow simmer with a bubble or 2 every few seconds. Cook for at least 3 hours stirring in 20-minute intervals. When the sauce gets dry from time-to-time add ½ cup of water to continue the cooking process and ensure the sauce does not burn.

- In the last half-hour of cooking, boil a pot of water and salt the water generously. Cook pappardelle al dente according to package instruction. Your pasta should have some bite to it but not be raw in the center. Save a tablespoon or 2 of the pasta water and set aside.
- When sauce is finished cooking, there should be no water left in the pot. The sauce should be shimmering and creamy from the fat and added at the beginning.
- Dump your pasta back into the pot add your pasta water, 1 tablespoon of butter, and pour over the cooked Bolognese sauce, toss to combine.

15. Grilled Lime Salmon With Avocado-Mango Salsa And Coconut Rice

Ingredients

Lime Salmon

- 4 6 Oz. skinless salmon fillets
- 3 Tbsp. olive oil, plus more for grill
- 2 Tsp. lime zest
- 3 Tbsp. fresh lime juice
- 3 Cloves garlic, crushed
- Salt and freshly ground black pepper, to taste

Coconut Rice

- 1½ Cups coconut water
- 1¼ Cups canned coconut milk
- 1½ Cups jasmine rice, rinsed well
- and drained well
- ½ Tsp. salt

Avocado-Mango Salsa

- 1 Large mango, peeled and diced
- ¾ Cup chopped red bell pepper (½ large)
- ¼ Cup chopped fresh cilantro
- 1/3 Cup chopped red onion, rinsed under water and drained
- 1 Large avocado, peeled and diced
- 1 Tbsp. fresh lime juice
- 1 Tbsp. olive oil
- 1 Tbsp. coconut water
- Salt and pepper, to taste

Directions

- For the Salmon:

In an 11x7-inch baking dish whisk together olive oil, lime zest, lime juice, garlic and season with salt and pepper to taste.

Place salmon in baking dish, cover and allow to marinate in refrigerator 15 to 30 minutes, then flip salmon to opposite side and allow to marinate 15 to 30 minutes longer. Preheat a grill over medium-high heat during last 10 minutes of marinating.

Brush grill grates with oil. Place salmon on grill and grill about 3 minutes per side or until just cooked through.

- For the Coconut Rice:

  While salmon is marinating, prepare coconut rice. In a medium saucepan bring coconut water, coconut milk, rice and salt to a full boil. Cover and simmer until liquid has mostly been absorbed about 20 minutes. Fluff with a fork, then let rest 5 minutes.

- For the Mango Avocado Salsa:

  While the rice is cooking, prepare salsa. In a medium bowl toss together mango, bell pepper, cilantro, red onion, avocado, lime juice, olive oil and coconut water. Season with salt and pepper to taste.

Serve salmon warm over coconut rice, and top with avocado mango salsa.

16. Vegetarian Kale And Beyond Meat Stir-Fry

Ingredients
- 3 Cloves of garlic
- 2 Pounds of lacinato kale
- 1 16 Oz. package of Beyond Meat
- 3 Tbsp. mirin (or any type of
- cooking wine)
- 1 ½ Tbsp. Korean bb☒ sauce
- 1 ½ Tsp. of chili oil
- 1 Tbsp. olive oil
- Cooked white or brown rice
- Sesame seeds (optional)

Directions
- Prep:

Mince garlic.

Wash and de-stem kale. Chop into 1 inch pieces.

Cook:

Heat up olive oil in a large skillet over medium heat. Add minced garlic and cook until fragrant, about 1 to 2 minutes.

Add package of Beyond Meat, breaking up into crumbles while sautéing/browning,

about 5 to 6 minutes.

Deglaze the pan with mirin or any cooking wine.

Add chopped kale, BBQ sauce, and chili oil, and mix together. Let that cook for about 3 to 4 minutes until kale is wilted.

Serve over white or brown rice.

Garnish with sesame seeds (optional).

17. Perfect Oatmeal

Ingredient

- 1 Cup whole oats
- (naturally gluten-free)
- 2 Cups water
- 1 Cup preferred plant-based milk
- (e.g.,almond, oat, coconut, etc.)
- 1 Tsp. seeds of choice (e.g.,chia,
- flax, pumpkin, hemp, etc.)
- 2 Servings preferred fruits
- (e.g.,banana, strawberries,
- blueberries, mango, peach, etc.)
- 2 Tsp. maple syrup
- Optional: 1 Tbsp. of raw nuts
- (e.g., shaved almond, pecans,
- walnuts)

Nutritionist says:

- For added protein, use oat milk, soy milk, or flax milk over the nut milks.
- Recommend about 1 cup total for the fruits.
- Fruits lend some sweetness, so feel free to omit the maple syrup asper taste preferences.
- Addition of raw nuts or can stir in 1 tbsp. of nut butters.

Instruction

- Add the oats and water to a pot on low to medium heat and slowly cook until water absorbs and oats become translucent (3 to 5 minutes).
- Optional: Dice and add banana to make it creamier and give it a banana bread flavor.
- Add the plant-based milk and stir until creamy (2 minutes).
- Add fruit, seeds, nuts and maple syrup.

18. Sweet Plantain Pancakes

Ingredients

- 1 Ripe plantain
- 1 Egg
- 1 or ½ Tbsp. unsweetened
- coconut flakes
- 1 or ½ Tbsp. chia seeds
- 1 Tsp. melted coconut oil
- ¼ Tsp. cinnamon

Directions

- Smash or blend sweet plantain.
- Add an egg and mix or blend together.
- Add coconut flakes, chia seeds, cinnamon, coconut oil and mix together.
- Cook on medium heat until bubbles form on the surface, then carefully flip and cook another 2 to 4 minutes.

- Serve with bluberries, strawberry, sliced almonds and maple syrup.

19. Roasted Salt Orange Fennel

Ingredients
- 2 Medium to large fennel bulbs,
- tops removed
- ½ Tsp. orange zest
- Juice from half an orange
- 1 Tbsp. lemon juice
- 2 to 3 Tbsp. olive oil

Directions
- Preheat oven to 400 degrees. Slice fennel bulbs in half and then into ¼ inch pieces. Toss in the orange juice and olive oil. Place in a casserole dish and bake for 20 to 25 minutes or until browned.

- Remove and stir in orange zest and lemon juice. Salt and pepper to taste.

20. Whole Roasted Cauliflower With Tahini Sauce

Ingredients
- 1 Medium cauliflower head
- 2 Tbsp. olive oil
- 2 Cloves garlic, minced
- ½ Cup of tahini paste
- ¼ Cup warm water
- ¼ Cup fresh lemon juice
- ½ Tsp. salt
- Optional: 1 tsp. harissa paste
- ½ Cup pepitas, raw (pumpkin seeds)
- Fresh herbs; about 2 tbsp. each of dill,basil, parsley

Directions

- Preheat your oven to 375 degrees. Line a baking sheet or shallow casserole dish with parchment paper or aluminum foil.
- Remove the leaves of the cauliflower, trim off the bottom stem, and wash thoroughlyPat dry.
- Rub the cauliflower all over generously with the olive oil.
- Place cauliflower stem side down on the baking sheet or casserole dish and place in a hot oven.
- Roast for 45 to 50 minutes until the cauliflower is fork-tender and lightly browned.
- While the cauliflower is roasting make your tahini sauce.
- Place a saute pan over medium-high heat with a light coating of olive oil.
- Add your crushed garlic and cook until soft and fragrant.

- Remove the pan from heat and add the tahini, warm water, garlic, lemon juice, salt, and harissa, if using. Whisk until well combined.
- Brush half of the tahini sauce all over the cauliflower.
- Cut cauliflower into six wedges and place on individual plates.
- Drizzle the remaining tahini sauce over the individual cauliflower servings.
- Sprinkle the chopped herbs and pepitas over the top and serve immediately.

21. Garlicky Green Beans

Ingredients
- 1 Pound of green beans, washed and trimmed
- 3 Cloves garlic, thinly sliced
- 2 Tbsp. olive oil
- 2 Tsp. coconut aminos

- A pinch of salt

Directions

- In a large pot, bring 6 cups of water to a boil. Add green beans and boil for about 3 to 5 minutes. Draingreen beans and place in a large bowl with filled with ice and water to stop the cooking. Heat oil in a pan over medium heat, add garlic and sauté for about 1 minute.
- Add the green beans and sauté for about 5 minutes. Stir in coconut aminos and cook for another 2 minutes. Turn off heat and add a pinch of salt and serve!

22. Roasted Turnips

Ingredients

- 2 Pounds of turnips
- 2 to 3 Tbsp. oil

- Salt and pepper to taste
- Optional: 2 tsp. Old Bay seasoning

Directions

- Preheat oven to 425 degrees.
- Cut the turnips in 1 to 2-inch pieces.
- Toss with olive oil and if using add the Old Bay and spread out onto a baking sheet lined with tin foil or parchment paper.
- Bake for about 20 minutes or until golden and crispy.
- Sprinkle with a pinch of salt and pepper to taste.

23. Anisette Cookies

Ingredients

- 1 Pound butter (softened)
- 2 Cups sugar
- 6 Heaping tbsp. sour cream

- 6 Cups sifted flour
- 2 Tsp. baking powder
- 2 Tsp. baking soda
- 2 Tsp. anise extract
- 4 Cups confectioner's sugar
- 2 to 3 Tsp. anise extract
- 6 Tbsp. milk
- Sprinkles

Directions

Making cookie dough:

- Mix all wet ingredients first in one bowl(butter, sour cream, eggs, and extract).
- In a second bowl, add and mix together all of the dry ingredients (sugar, flour, baking soda and powder).
- While mixer or food processor is on, add flour mixture slowly to the wet ingredients.

- Using two pieces of wax paper, create a kneading area for the dough. Sprinkle flour on wax paper andhands. Continue to flour hands if they feel sticky. Divide dough into 4 parts.
- Knead each part and roll into 4 balls. Place in dry bowl and cover with wax paper or throw each ball into a ziploc bag.
- Refrigerate for several hours or overnight. Some can be frozen.

Baking cookies:

- Grease and flour cookie sheet. Take out 1 ball of dough at a time, and pinch off a little dough. Roll into 1" balls and place on cookie sheet.
- Bake for about 8-10 mins or until light golden brown along bottom edges. Let cook for at least 30 mins.

Icing and glazing cookies:

- Mix powdered sugar, extract and milk together until loose consistency of a pudding before it sets. Add more powdered sugar to thicken if necessary.
- Dip each cookie in mixture and place onwax paper.
- Sprinkle with sprinkles.
- Store in airtight container

24. Apple spice hemp muffins

Ingredients

- 1 ½ Cups whole-grain spelt flour
- 1 Cup oat flour
- ¾ Cup hemp seeds
- 1 ½ to 2 Tsp. cinnamon
- ¼ Tsp. salt
- ¼ Tsp. cardamom ground or nutmeg
- 2 Tsp. baking powder

- ½ Tsp. baking soda
- 1 Cup unsweetened organic applesauce
- ¾ Cup plain or vanilla nondairy milk
- ½ Cup pure maple syrup
- 1 ½ Tsp. vanilla extract
- 1/3 Cup raisins – or substitute dark vegan
- chocolate chips

Optional (makes them taste like morning glory muffins):

- 1/3 Cup grated apple
- 1/3 Cup grated carrot

Directions

- Preheat oven to 350 degrees.
- In a large bowl combine the flours, hemp seeds, cinnamon, salt, cardamon, baking powder and baking soda, i.e. all the dry ingredients, and mix well to combine fully.

- In a smaller bowl mix all the wet ingredients applesauce, milk, maple syrup, vanilla extract then add the raisins and, if using, the apple and carrots and mix well.
- Fold the wet mixture into the dry one until just combined.
- Spoon into cupcake liners.
- Bake for 25 minutes until a toothpick inserted in the center comes out clean.

25. Ginger Tumeric Tea

This tea is not only delicious but also aids in reducing inflammation

Ingredient
- 8 oz boiling water
- 1 tsp. fresh turmeric root, grated (1/3 tsp. if using dried)

- 1 tsp. fresh ginger root, grated (1/3 tsp. if using dried)
- 1 tsp. coconut oil
- Honey to taste, optional

- Fresh lemon wedge, optional
- Combine all ingredients.

26. Berry-Banana Smoothie

This delicious smoothie is great for lupus patients experiencing fatigue but will also help prevent bone loss and cardiovascular disease.

Ingredients
- 1 cup of low-fat yogurt (any flavor)
- 1/2 cup of round oat cereal (i.e. Cheerios)
- 2 tablespoons ground flax-seed or flax-seed meal

- 1/2 cup fresh strawberry halves or raspberries, or frozen whole strawberries
- 1/2 cup skim milk or vanilla Rice Drink (non-dairy beverage)
- 1/2 banana

Directions

- Place all ingredients in blender. Cover and blend on high speed 10 seconds; stop blender to scrape sides. Cover and blend about 20 seconds longer or until smooth.
- Pour mixture into glasses. Serve immediately.

27. Salmon Teriyaki

This is a simple, yet healthy way to prepare salmon. Serve salmon with steamed broccoli and brown rice.

Ingredients

- 8 oz salmon filet
- ¾ cup thawed pineapple juice concentrate
- 1 Tbsp chopped fresh ginger
- 1 Tbsp chopped garlic
- 3 Tbsp low sodium organic soy sauce
- 1 Tbsp rice vinegar

Directions

- Divide the salmon into two 4 oz portions.
- Combine the pineapple juice concentration, rice vinegar, soy sauce, garlic and ginger in a small bowl.
- In a non-stick skillet, over medium-high heat, brown the salmon filets, about 3 minutes each side.
- Pour half the teriyaki sauce over the salmon in the skillet and cook for an additional 5 minutes or until the salmon is cooked through.

- Serve with the remaining teriyaki sauce.
- Divide the salmon into two 4 oz portions.Combine the pineapple juice concentration, rice vinegar, soy sauce, garlic and ginger in a small bowl.In a non-stick skillet, over medium-high heat, brown the salmon filets, about 3 minutes each side.Pour half the teriyaki sauce over the salmon in the skillet and cook for an additional 5 minutes or until the salmon is cooked through.Serve with the remaining teriyaki sauce.

28. Sunny Juice

A naturally sweet and low-glycemic raw, veggie juice that's packed with ingredients to boost your mood, heart health, improve your blood pressure, and ensure optimal digestion of nutrients!

Ingredients

- 1 head of organic romaine lettuce, washed or 1 bunch of organic kale
- 1 organic lemon
- 1 large organic carrot, peeled
- 2 stalks of organic celery
- 1 one-inch knob of ginger root
- 1/2 an organic cucumber (or zucchini)
- (optional): 1/4-1/2 a green apple (or a leftover apple core)

Method

- Add all the ingredients to the juicer in the order listed and juice.
- Pour the juice over a glass of ice for a nice and chilled juice, and enjoy!
- Clean the juicer immediately after (this is much easier to do right now than later). Let the juicer parts dry well and put away for tomorrow.

29. Green Funnel Lime Juice

Fennel is a great ingredient for a green juice, as it offers a subtle distinct mild licorice flavor and is very light on the calories. Nutritionally, it's a great source of minerals such as calcium and potassium and also contains folate and vitamin C. This low-sugar juice has great flavor, especially if you add the fennel leaves.

Ingredients
- 1 fennel bulb
- 1 large green apple
- 2 large celery sticks
- 1 Lebanese cucumber
- 1 lime

Method
- Wash, scrub and chop the produce

- Juice & enjoy with ice!

30. Pineapple Green Tea Juice

Ingredients
- ¼ pineapple
- 1 lemon
- 1 cup of cooled green tea

Method
- Peel the pineapple and scrub the lemon (peeling the lemon is optional).
- Juice pineapple and lemon through a juicer.
- Prepare the green tea and allow to cool.
- Combine the pineapple and lemon juice with the green tea.
- Add ice and enjoy!

Printed in Great Britain
by Amazon

26152547R00050